The Gift of Remission

A JOURNEY INTO MULTIPLE SCLEROSIS AND BACK AGAIN

LINDA LAND

Outskirts Press, Inc
Denver, Colorado

The Gift of Remission
A Journey Into Multiple Sclerosis and Back Again

V3.0

Photographic Artist:
Desirée Suchy
http://www.photographybydesiree.com

Cover and Interior Designer:
Launie Perry
red letter creative

Outskirts Press, Inc.
http://www.outskirtspress.com

ISBN: 978-1-4327-4216-4

PRINTED IN THE UNITED STATES OF AMERICA

Dedicated to those who have
the creativity and courage
to expand our thinking

CONTENTS

FOREWORD

I MET LINDA LAND A FEW YEARS ago when she contacted me about the manuscript that would become this book. As I began to read her personal odyssey into the terrible world that is multiple sclerosis, I was immediately drawn to the message of hope and optimism she had so carefully crafted in this uplifting and wonderful human story of trial, tribulation, and eventual triumph over this crippling and fatal disease. I consider it a privilege to be one of the first people to have read this masterful anecdote about one person's victory over multiple sclerosis through diet.

This book is not a scientific treatise on how or why diet may be involved in the pathogenesis of multiple sclerosis, but rather a compelling narrative of how Linda's husband—

and others like him—collectively arrived at a successful dietary strategy to treat multiple sclerosis. I endorse this book because I believe the scientific literature increasingly supports the notion that diet is one of the most important environmental factors responsible for eliciting multiple sclerosis in genetically susceptible individuals.

Numerous human clinical studies reveal that increased intestinal permeability (commonly called "leaky gut") frequently precedes the development of symptoms in many autoimmune diseases, including multiple sclerosis. It is thought that resident gut bacteria that normally would not have access to the bloodstream and the immune system gain entry when the gut becomes "leaky." Common foods such as wheat, beans, legumes, dairy products, egg whites and certain members of the nightshade family contain so-called "anti-nutrients" that increase intestinal permeability and allow gut bacteria and their by-products to continually stimulate the immune system. Normally, in people who don't develop multiple sclerosis, this continual stimulation results in "oral tolerance." Unfortunately, oral tolerance is abrogated in multiple sclerosis patients because of their genetic susceptibility (MHC haplotype) to the disease. Additionally, some of the same foods that promote a "leaky gut" also contain other anti-nutrients, known as "adjuvants," which are routinely used in vaccines to elicit powerful responses by the immune system. In effect, multiple sclerosis patients are unknowingly vaccinating themselves against their own tissues through a process called "molecular mimicry" caused by anti-nutrients found in everyday foods. By eliminating these foods and restoring the gut barrier, it is possible to calm the immune system and lessen or eliminate symptoms, particularly if the disease is caught in its early stages.

Science and medicine are not static processes. They dynamically change as new information replaces yesterday's "truths." The past dogma was that diet had little to do with multiple sclerosis. However, in large human networks, people frequently arrive at correct solutions to complex problems before science can explain the underlying mechanisms. I believe that such is the case for multiple sclerosis and diet. Linda and others like her have found a dietary solution to the disease, and an emerging body of scientific evidence suggests that they were right all along.

Loren Cordain, Ph.D.

Professor, Human and Environmental Sciences
Colorado State University
Fort Collins, Colorado
February 5, 2009

PREFACE

IN 1980, MY HUSBAND AND I WERE handed an amazing gift of information that helped my husband recover from multiple sclerosis, an autoimmune disease. At the time, we didn't know why the suggested steps worked; we were simply grateful they facilitated the full remission. However, concerned about the genetic susceptibility of our children, we continued to watch for links between the nutritional information we followed and scientific research results. Now that cutting-edge, validating research is available. It's our intention, first of all, to convey this message of hope and healing to those who are dealing with an autoimmune disease and need the information immediately. Second, we'd like to raise the awareness of those who don't even realize they are setting themselves up for a devastating illness. It's time to pass along the gift to as many people as possible.

PROLOGUE

Spring 2004

CRISP MORNING SUNLIGHT spilled through the oversized, eastern window in the unfinished basement. I surveyed my self-imposed reorganizing project and smiled. The portion completed was finally beginning to outweigh that yet to sort. At one end of the room was a collection of mismatched, crumple-edged boxes labeled and relabeled with black and blue markers. At the opposite end were neatly stacked, plastic storage containers with matching lids. Attached to the end of each container was a clear pocket holding an index card that carefully listed the contents within.

I opened the window a few inches to freshen the air and then set my mug of tea where it would remain safely out of the way of the expected paper-strewn mess. Although I had done most of the original packing and labeling, with the distancing of time, each box held surprises.

With practiced movements, I opened another dog-eared, cardboard mystery. Tossing the crumpled top layers of paper aside, I began to free objects from their padded and wedged confinement. I grabbed one item after another from the box, discarding the protective, yellowed newsprint. A quick judgment determined each object's destination, until my hand emerged clutching the handle of a cane that hadn't been needed for years. I remembered quite vividly my thoughts when I packed it the last time, and a sense of gratitude swept over me.

I automatically reached for my tea, nesting the bottom of the mug in my left hand as I grasped the handle with my right. I took a distracted sip as I pondered my options for this familiar object. My eyes wandered to the light pouring through the window as my thoughts drifted to a time and place I hadn't visited for a long time.

CHAPTER 1: SYMPTOMS

Fall 1979

I LEANED AGAINST THE EDGE of the kitchen counter, soaking in the morning's milky haze as my fingers absorbed the warmth of my cradled teacup. Looking through the open window, I unwrapped the package of this new day, filling my senses with quiet anticipation. I playfully imagined autumn casually draping her favorite fabrics over the golf-course landscape beyond. Paisley patterns of sage green, crimson red, and cinnamon orange festooned red oaks and sugar maples. Beyond the golf course lay a golden corduroy of harvested wheat stubble.

The quiet calm of the haze outside began to lift as activity inside the house gained momentum. Three-year-old twins Todd and Ryan spilled their combined morning exuberance into the kitchen. I quickly set my cup of tea safely on the counter before four arms encircled my legs. Bending down, I gathered both boys into my arms to return their enthusiastic hugs. Soon, echoing calls of "Daddy, Daddy!" heralded Rich and Duffer's return from an early morning jog on the golf course. I was pleased to see that my husband, Rich, had managed to navigate our golden retriever around the water hazards this morning as he let the tail-wagging protector into the house to check on her self-proclaimed twin charges. They each gave her a hug before Rich scooped them into his arms, laughing warmly as he greeted each. I laughed with them, and then turned my attention to breakfast and the other morning routines.

A little while later, Rich, freshly showered and dressed, called to me from the hallway. "I'll be back in a few minutes," he said. "I need to check on the painter who's supposed to be at the office this morning for some touch-up work. It shouldn't take too long, and then I'll be back to play with the boys. We'll probably need to head to the game on the early side. They're expecting quite a crowd today."

I relished the fact that the construction of Rich's new dental office building was complete. The design and construction stages had consumed so much of his time. For months I had observed his difficult juggling of schedules to keep up with the needs of his patients, his construction project, and his family. His generous nature had him stretched, trampoline-thin, in many directions. I loved Saturdays when he was not working, especially Saturday game days.

Fall football-game days in Lawrence, Kansas had their own exciting rhythm. Field after field of marching golden cornstalks with feathery plumes escorted the opposing team and fans into town. Raucous band tunes were carried in the breeze and spun to the ground on the backs of playful leaves. Students and alumni paraded along with new and old friends, scattering the fallen leaves to reveal undulating mounds of uneven bricks on the sidewalks winding their way toward the stadium. Excited conversations mixed with mellow sunshine. Rich and I, hand in hand, joined in the game day fall fun.

It all seemed so perfect—until Rich released his left hand and repositioned me to his right side. I immediately understood the significance of the move, and an anxious expression replaced my smile. "Will you call the doctor?" I asked pointedly.

"I will if it doesn't improve," Rich responded in a forced yet casual manner. His concern appeared to be growing with mine. Something was wrong with his left arm.

CHAPTER 2: PROGRESSION

Winter 1979-80

I SHIVERED, TIGHTLY GRIPPED my tea mug, and stepped back from the window. Ice etched brittle patterns on the windowpanes and created treacherous walking and driving. I thought Rich and I might be walking on black ice as well. The intermittent numbness in Rich's left arm continued. With my concerned prompting, he eventually sought an appointment with his internist.

The visit with Rich's doctor left many questions unanswered. Although the doctor couldn't completely rule out a connection with heart disease, he thought it unlikely. He did think it might have something to do with the amount of stress that Rich was experiencing and suggested finding ways to reduce the stress.

We decided that a long-overdue vacation might be the perfect way for Rich to relax. If the problem was heart- or stress-related, he needed a break from his daily routine. In mid-February, we chose a coastal retreat where we could wander aimlessly along the beach and enjoy uninterrupted time. It was a welcome change of pace for both of us, but it didn't remedy the numbness in Rich's arm.

Upon our return, the internist ordered a complete series of testing. Rich hated the time involved with the testing, but as other symptoms were beginning to crop up, he needed to know what was going on. At times he had difficulty with his vision, unexplained headaches and balance issues, and the numbness in his left arm had moved into his hand. As someone whose livelihood depended entirely on his hands, Rich needed answers right away.

But answers were not readily available. The

initial tests were inconclusive, so more in-depth testing was recommended. Rich had no choice but to endure another round of poking and probing, yet definitive conclusions still could not be drawn. During this time, Rich vacillated between frustrated anger directed at his body and total denial that there was anything seriously wrong. After more than a month of fruitless testing, one physician friend suggested the name of a disease that might be causing the symptoms. He said it was a "garbage can diagnosis," because there was no way to test for it directly. It was only diagnosed as a possibility if all the testing did not conclusively lead in another direction. The disease was called MS, or multiple sclerosis.

Rich and I were stunned. We each had known someone who had been debilitated by MS, and those mental pictures were far from the successful future we had imagined for ourselves. As we sought advice within the medical community about our options, the recurring answer from the physicians was "nothing." Just as there was no definitive test for the disease, there was also no cure.

Rich and I felt as though we had been racing along, achieving our dream, when suddenly and inexplicably, the engine had shut down. It was as if our car had coasted to the pit lane and was left stranded as our vision raced on without us.

We shared anger. How could this garbage disease unwind all that we had worked so hard to create? We had invested so much time, expense, and energy in Rich's training, building the clinic, and establishing trust with his patients. We couldn't just give it all up without a fight. But what was our opponent? How would we fight a disease with no cure, a disease with a list of symptoms that could make it impossible for Rich to continue his dental practice?

At first it seemed too incredible to consider. Our initial outrage, however, steadily transformed into a sense of resolve as Rich's health progressively deteriorated. With each passing week, he increasingly had to postpone treatments or move procedures to the other dentists in the practice. He continued to experience intermittent numbness in the fingers of his left hand, blurred vision, and headaches. He couldn't be certain he would be able to perform with the high level of precision his work demanded. The stress of working too much and too many hours was being replaced by the stress associated with the inability to work enough.

And so, Rich began the unthinkable process of turning his practice over to the other dentists in the building. The state of his health had made the decision for him. The other dentists were hopeful Rich would stay on and continue to do what he could, but Rich found it emotionally difficult to be a part of the practice while physically functioning at a weakened level. His energy and drive had been the key elements in creating his successful practice. Now Rich knew he had to detach while he still had enough energy to facilitate a smooth transition for his patients.

Rich and I knew our financial situation was temporarily stable, thanks to our shared insistence on saving. Because we were self-employed, we had set aside enough money to cover our expenses for six months in case of an emergency. We also had the funds we had been saving for remodeling our home—money that could carry us for another six months. It was an incredible safety net.

The wild card was the eventual impact of the disabilities. We did not know what Rich would be capable of doing. I briefly considered returning to teaching in the fall, but my position on the subject changed with the discovery that I was expecting another baby. Even though our vacation to the coast hadn't improved Rich's condition, the relaxed time together had brought about the unplanned pregnancy.

I waited to tell Rich about the baby until it was absolutely confirmed. I felt that every child was a precious gift, but the timing of this gift seemed to reach the ridiculous realm.

When I told Rich, the enormous absurdity of the situation forced us past regret, and we firmly resolved to make the most of the situation. We laughed at the circumstances with tears streaming down our faces. How could such careful planners let everything get so totally out of control?

For the first time, we stopped talking about how to sandbag the dam and began talking instead about how to survive the imminent flood. We began to openly acknowledge that the only control we had over these events was the manner in which we chose to handle them. We could not allow these challenges to break our spirits. We had to work together to stay positive and keep our sense of humor. It was our attitude that would make the only difference. The value-center messages in our minds assured us there were hidden windows of opportunity to be discovered.

CHAPTER 3: GUIDANCE

Spring 1980

SPRING'S EXPANSIVE ENERGY and colorful palette replaced winter's stale chill. Chartreuse blades of grass popped out of the tawny, matted golf-course fairways. Jonquils lined our patio, and creamy buds burst open on our tulip trees. Warm breezes infused me with sweet-scented, renewed spirit.

I knew Rich and I couldn't allow our sidetracked dreams to keep us in a state of inactivity for very long. We had to focus on recreating and repositioning our lives, using our safety net of funds to facilitate the action. We needed to act while we still had some control.

Both Rich and I wanted to take charge of our thoughts and actions, but we were torn among so many unknowns. We had, up to this point, boldly planned adventures and dreams in great detail, feeling confident in our ability to fulfill them. Now that bold certainty was faltering.

I tried to get an inward sense of direction while outwardly attempting to keep a normal routine for the twins. I knew Todd and Ryan mirrored my attitude, so I worked extra hard to be positive and calm around them. I also kept the twins and myself involved in our regular activities as much as possible while Rich and I decided how to proceed.

One spring morning, I dropped Todd and Ryan off at one of their favorite activities, an art class for three-year-olds hosted by Parks and Recreation. I greeted and visited briefly with a friend as the eager young artists embarked on another messy painting project. I intended to use the forty-five minutes to run an errand, but I decided instead to leave the car parked where it was, and I began to walk.

It was the first time in days that I had been

alone. As I walked, I was barely aware of the lovely historic houses I passed or of the miniature yellow-green foliage and pastel shades of early spring flowers. I hardly noticed the sidewalk beneath my feet. The encounter with my friend had unnerved me. I was finding it harder and harder to maintain a stoic facade when I answered questions about Rich's health. Tears fell unnoticed onto my cheeks.

Hammering waves of emotion rammed into me, eroding the footing of my precarious balance. One unsettling wave tore at the core message that I was capable of handling any situation. I felt anything *but* capable as I helplessly watched Rich's health deteriorate with each day. Another toppling wave of fearful unknowns caught me off-center as I struggled to recover from the last churning wave. I knew I should take one moment at a time, making it the best that I could, yet each unknown undermined my ability to stay in the moment.

The unknowns were like sharp thorns

pricking my heart and seeping my energy away. The tears continued to surface as my heart silently cried for help. My sense of self-preservation instinctively turned my thoughts toward God, my life's source. Usually my prayers were calm streams of grateful thought or sourcing of energy that gently surfaced and conversed like a quiet brook meanders through a wide meadow of possibilities. But this prayer surged with the intensity of a spring-swollen river cutting and overflowing its banks. Every part of my being focused as I handed our situation to God and trusted that wisdom and guidance would be handed back to me.

I wasn't sure how long I'd been standing beneath the dappled, leafy canopy of the elder oak. I felt slightly disoriented as my senses reawakened to my surroundings. Suddenly aware of the tears that had spilled down my face, I swept my fingers quickly across my cheeks. Glancing at my watch, I was relieved to discover that the art class would not end for another ten minutes. I said a silent *thank you* to God, as I always did whenever something went well, but then I found myself repeating it over and over. This time I was saying it with much more fervor for the magnitude of the guidance and wisdom that I knew was forth-coming.

A few days later, the guidance began. It was not in the form of something bold and shouted, but rather in subtle whispers of ideas. Rich was in front of the house putting the trash can out for the next morning collection. When he had not returned after several minutes, I observed from the window that he was having a conversation with the passengers of a car that was parked at the bottom of the driveway.

When Rich came back inside, I curiously asked, "Who were you visiting with?"

Rich replied, "They were just some people who were looking at a couple of houses for sale in the area. They wanted to get a feel for the neighborhood. Nice people."

I went back to what I'd been doing, and then, without any fanfare, the thoughts began to take voice in my mind. I looked at Rich and asked abruptly, "Did you say anything to them about our house maybe being for sale?"

Rich returned my gaze and said, "No, I didn't know it *was* for sale. When did we get to that point?" He seemed slightly annoyed, as though we'd been walking side by side, and now, all of a sudden, I was several strides ahead of him.

He was right. We had not talked about selling the house. We had, however, discussed the limitations of our two-story house if Rich's legs deteriorated. His left leg had already begun to have moments of weakness. My parents had also encouraged us to move closer to them, so they could help with the twins and the baby should I decide to return to teaching right away. The offer of assistance was certainly welcome, but it meant completely uprooting to another city in another state. Two years ago, my parents had moved from central Kansas to Colorado Springs, Colorado. Rich and I loved our little college town, but we considered the suggestion. If this dream was ending, maybe it would be easier and wiser to begin another dream in another place. This town would hold constant reminders of our former life.

I began again, more cautiously, "Well, if we *were* to decide to move closer to my parents and *did* decide to sell this house, do you think those people might be interested in knowing that it's for sale?"

Rich appeared to weigh the question for a moment before answering. "They did say several times, come to think of it, how much they liked our house and how it was obvious that we worked hard to take good care of it and the yard."

"Do you have any idea how we'd be able to get in touch with them again, *if* we wanted to?" I questioned with continued caution.

"The man said they were moving here so

he could take a position in the Engineering Department at the university," Rich replied. "You know, the professor who sits beside us at the football games is part of the Engineering School faculty. He'd probably be able to find out who's been hired and how to contact him. Seems like a real long shot though..."

"Hmm. Probably," I agreed. "Well, let's think about it." I let the subject drop.

We did continue to think about it, off and on, during the next day and into the weekend. Rich mentioned the topic again on Sunday evening. "I think I'll give the professor a call tomorrow and see if he might know how to get in touch with those people," he said.

The next evening, upon arriving home from work, Rich walked into the backyard. Duffer was the first to greet him, with her whole body wagging. Todd and Ryan engulfed him next with their hugs and laughter, but soon returned to their game of clubbing oversized plastic balls with yellow plastic bats. Rich kissed me and settled in next to me at the patio table as long rays of early-evening, mellow sunlight backlit our family gathering and the sleepy golf course beyond.

I searched Rich's face for information. His increasing fatigue had darkened the areas beneath his eyes, and now he looked especially exhausted. I inquired about his day. He rested a heavy head on one hand and allowed the events to trickle out. He said that he hadn't felt well enough to do anything other than minor exams and had to reschedule more difficult procedures since he couldn't trust his hands with the high-speed equipment. As he said this, I could sense a surge of anger welling up inside him, followed by the emotional bruising of guilt. He said he couldn't believe his body was creating so much turmoil for our family. He had never before experienced a time when he did not feel that he was in control. His perception had always been that if he wanted something, he just had to work hard enough to get it or accomplish whatever it was. If it meant working harder or working longer, Rich had always been able to create whatever he desired. But now his belief statement was in direct conflict with his body's condition. He felt as if the rules of the game had changed on him; just when Rich thought he was winning, he was about to lose everything he had worked so hard to achieve.

Rich stretched and straightened his back a little, looking over the serene calm of the golf course. For the hundredth time, Rich willed the weakening thoughts of guilt out of his mind. He would not allow himself to be caught up in such useless and wasteful thinking. He told me that even while some of his perceptions were jamming, the survival thoughts were taking over. He said he did not want to leave this dream anymore than I did, but it seemed that both of us were being led in another direction.

"So, I called the professor," Rich said, exhaustion evident in his clipped tone. "I explained the situation to him as briefly as possible. He was very kind and quickly called back after locating the name and phone number of the incoming engineering instructor. But," Rich continued, "the professor also found out that they flew back yesterday to their home on the east coast."

"Well, I wonder if they bought one of the other houses. Guess we won't know unless we call them," I said in a matter-of-fact manner.

"Call them! They're halfway across the country!" Rich said incredulously. He seemed to think it acceptable to contact the people while they were still in town, but this was carrying it too far. "What would I say to them?" he continued. "Hey, I'm the guy you talked with beside the trash can, and I was just wondering if you might want to come back and check out my house?"

I laughed and agreed it sounded preposterous, but I persisted. "Well, who cares how it sounds! We'll never know if they bought something else unless we call them. And, what if they didn't? Maybe they would love to buy our house. We should at least let them know that we're considering selling."

Rich said that he still thought it was a long shot, but he agreed to call them while I started the boys' evening ritual of a bath followed by story time. I was halfway through the bathing process when Rich walked in with a surprised expression on his face.

"They're interested," he stated with overtones of dismay in his voice. "I can't believe it. They left town without making an offer on any of the houses because they just didn't find what they really wanted. And here's the kicker. They're going to contact their relatives who live about thirty minutes from here to see if they'd be willing to come over and look at the inside of our house. Anyway, I guess we'll be hearing from them." He was clearly baffled by the sheer coincidence of it all.

Moments later, Rich settled into our oversized oak rocker for the evening picture book story session. Immediately, the rocker was overflowing with two freshly bathed, pajama-clad boys and one very large Richard Scarry picture book. The twins adored the identification game they played every evening and were soon giggling over the process. Rich had not been certain of his left arm and hand throughout the day, so he concentrated on holding the book in his right hand and was soon caught up in the boys' enthusiasm.

I wandered off, welcoming a few moments to myself as I silently voiced a thank you. I did not feel nearly as surprised as Rich did about the people wanting to see our house. Instead, I felt a warm sense of peaceful gratitude and a sense that this was part of God's plan. I had no idea how things would play out, but I felt that we needed to be open to whatever began to materialize.

When the phone rang the next morning, it took me a few seconds to register the significance of the caller's name. "Why, yes," I said. "Tomorrow afternoon will be just fine. I'll look forward to meeting you." I put the phone down. A look of apprehension appeared momentarily on my face as I thought *That was awfully fast.* But then the reality of having the house ready to show the next day set in as I looked at the toy-strewn family room. "Guess we'll have to be fast, too," I said to the twins as I enlisted their help.

The next two weeks went warp speed for Rich and me. The relatives took photos of the house to send to the prospective buyers. Within a week, an offer had been made. And, by the end of the second week, all of the details had been worked out. The new owners wanted possession by July.

It was as if the uncertainty of whether or not to leave had been settled for us by the whirlwind events of selling the house. In fact, when all the negotiations were complete, Rich and I realized that the finality of the sale left no doubt about our decision. We were leaving.

Rich and I spent a couple of days adjusting to the decision we knew we had made. Somehow, though, it felt like the decision had been made for us. We talked of returning if Rich's health improved. We felt fortunate to move at a good time for my pregnancy. We knew it would be nice for the twins to be near their grandparents. We did not talk about how hard it would be to leave our friends and Rich's patients. We both felt that in order to turn this challenge into an opportunity, there was no time or energy for dwelling on our losses. We had to focus on moving forward and making the best of our unknown future.

I watched Rich struggle to turn his patients over to his partners. The days he did not feel capable of working began to equal or outnumber the ones in which he felt up to the task. I realized I had to assume responsibility for getting us moved. I wasn't exactly sure how to proceed, but after a few phone calls, I'd contacted three different moving companies to obtain bids on the move. And, with a little more organizing, I set up travel arrangements for the twins and myself for a house-hunting trip near my parents.

I had my hands full while traveling with Todd and Ryan. Going anywhere with the twins was like tagging along beside a lively parade.

They always had a great time, no matter what they were doing, and bystanders were naturally attracted to the good-natured duo. My role was to keep the parade headed in the right direction and its noise level muted.

After settling the twins with my parents, knowing they would be well cared for and entertained, I began looking for a new home. Before I left, Rich and I agreed that we hoped I would be able to find something affordable in the vicinity of my parents' home and on one level, in case Rich's mobility became progressively debilitated. It wasn't until the end of the second day looking at houses that I realized the limiting extent of our conditions. So far, nothing had even come close to meeting all our requirements.

On the third morning, I tried not to be discouraged by the two fruitless days as I slid into the front seat next to my real estate agent. We drove around the corner from my parents' home and simultaneously spotted a new "For Sale" sign in a yard. The house was ranch style, and the listing agency was the same as my real estate agent's. Within minutes we had arranged to see the house, and once inside, I knew it was perfect. I had envisioned sending photos to Rich, as our buyers had done, but I quickly realized there wouldn't be time for that sort of luxury. Since this house met all our conditions, I phoned Rich to get his approval and made an offer. By the end of the day, we had a contract in hand and would take possession on the first of July.

I really hadn't known what to expect when I embarked on the house-hunting venture. But even my most idyllic dreams couldn't have created an easier process. Once again, I felt as though I were being gently escorted through the challenges. Usually I required considerable time to weigh all my options. To my amazement, however, I felt comfortably strong and capable of making timely decisions. I knew I wasn't doing this alone. I knew without a doubt that a greater power was caring for me and allowing everything to fall into place. I was awestruck by the ease. God was handling it. Windows were opening.

CHAPTER 4: WISDOM

Summer 1980

I RESTED MY BACK AGAINST the cluttered kitchen countertop, cradled my arms around my expanding belly, and squinted into the simmering western sunlight. Vivid black-eyed Susans and orange-red geraniums in terracotta pots lazed on our porch steps, while swallows swooped under the eaves to untidy nests of mud and straw. Locusts wove discordant concerts with two-toned droning.

Within the welcome cool of the air conditioning, I tackled the household packing slowly and methodically, knowing that I still had three weeks to accomplish the task. I was relieved when the activities that the twins and I had been involved in throughout the spring took a summer break. My answers to concerned queries about Rich's health had become almost robotic. I could hear myself repeating, "No, the doctors aren't really sure what it is, although they suspect it might be MS. Yes, we've decided to move closer to family, at least until we know how this all sorts out." I did not even realize how mechanical my responses had become until the first Sunday in June.

It was a sunny day, and I felt drawn outside of the private shelter created by my solitary packing task. Even though Rich didn't feel up to attending church, I put the top down on the convertible, buckled the twins in the back seat, and followed the familiar route. Sunshine warmed the early morning air as the convertible ambled along, and windswept tendrils of hair tickled our necks.

Todd and Ryan scrambled up the steps ahead of me. They happily joined friends in the preschool area, while I slipped quietly into a side pew in the sanctuary. I rarely went to church without Rich and missed leaning into his shoulder during the service. I forced my mind to focus instead on the gleaming dark wood, the kaleidoscope of colors streaming through stained-glass windows, the spoken and sung words. I was beginning to ready myself to leave as the congregation sang together at the end of the service when the full impact of the hymn caught in my throat.

I had comfortably sung those words countless times before, but this time tears welled in my eyes as I fought to regain my composure. I was caught with my guard down, and the song's meaning bit into me. "Until we meet again..." conjured renewed uncertainties as the unknown pulled Rich and me away from our friends and all we knew.

Clenching my teeth to force the tears away, I quickly made my way up the stairs to collect the twins. I hoped to slip out a side door, but I suddenly found myself surrounded once again by concerned questions. I tried to recall my rote answers and steady my presence, even though internally I was falling apart. Just as my tears were welling up again, a friend recognized the panic in my eyes and took charge. She ushered the twins and me toward the door, all the while fending off questions with soothing responses.

As I escaped into the sunlight, I recognized a reflection of my own sadness in the eyes of my friend. I could not trust my voice to communicate my appreciation, but my friend heard anyway. I gathered the twins' hands in mine and retreated.

As we walked toward the car, I became fully aware of how negligent I had been in not realizing how difficult it would be to leave our friends. Things left unsaid don't go away; they in fact have a way of biting harder when they finally surface. They wait for an unexpected, vulnerable moment to claim space and time. If Rich and I had given voice to this aspect of our leaving, or if I had not suppressed my feelings with robotic responses, I would have been more prepared for this heartfelt sting.

Rich was also bearing the brunt of things left unsaid. As easy as the house sale and purchase process had been, detaching from the dental practice was anything but easy. When we set up the practice, the disability provision documents appeared so black and white. Now those seemingly well-defined edges were full of value variances, making the process incredibly difficult for everyone involved. Rich's energy lagged with each frustrating gray area until the confusing process finally concluded.

I felt his hardest moments with him. As Rich closed the door to his office, we both knew that he was probably closing this part of his life altogether. He and his partners attempted to put in return stipulations in case his health recovered, but the whole exercise was as vague as the unknowns of the illness. Four years of dental school, two years of practicing in the army, and five years of private practice now lay behind a closed door. Rich fought to subdue the anger-filled sadness that boiled within him as he walked away.

The last week of June brought unusually hot weather. Our air-conditioner compressor hummed continually. The golf-course fairways and neighborhood lawns quickly traded their lush, emerald carpets for sprinkler patterns surrounded by parched brown perimeters.

Rich and I worked together to finish packing before the movers arrived. Even though we were glad to be occupied inside, where it was pleasantly cool, we found ourselves struggling on an emotional rollercoaster. But this time we recognized the symptoms, and as soon as one of us began to mentally stagger downward, the other worked to divert the fall and buoy the spirits. It was at this time, too, that friends made the biggest difference.

Most of our friends understood and supported the decision to move to Colorado during this time of unraveling, and it was the small, simple gestures from these friends that helped us through those last few days. One friend arrived with a wheat-engraved, locally made ceramic bowl filled with fresh strawberries. Another brought a butterfly magnet for our next refrigerator door. Others came by to visit or to help entertain the twins. Finally, though, the door to the house was locked and the moving van door latched shut.

Upon our arrival in Colorado Springs, it was once again the small, welcoming gestures of new neighbors that made all the difference. One neighbor pulled a red wagon down the sidewalk carrying her preschooler, who was steadying a pitcher of lemonade and a plate of cookies. Another neighbor arrived with flowers and an invitation for the twins to play with her young children. Because my parents were part of this neighborhood, it seemed that everyone understood the circumstances of the move and tactfully steered away from prying questions. Most were respectful of our privacy, but others were young professionals who identified with the tremendous upheaval and untimely nature of this move.

We unpacked quickly, thanks to the extra hands and energy of my parents, Virginia and Marvin. When my parents weren't assisting me, they kept the twins entertained so I could get more done. I appreciated all the help, and I felt a renewed energy, sustained by the cooler mountain air. I hoped it would be a similar tonic for Rich.

As the weeks passed, the cool temperatures of the foothill city felt better to Rich, but the climate wasn't improving his symptoms. He was experiencing more problems with his vision and continued weakening of the left side of his body. He reluctantly started to rely on a cane for stability. Just nine months ago, Rich had been jogging around the perimeter of the golf course, and now it could be a struggle to stay upright. He tried to keep his sense of humor, to joke about the spills and awkward movements.

Both Rich and I knew we needed to focus on our visions for the future rather than dwell on our fears. However, he seemed to realize I was having as hard a time envisioning a positive outcome as he was, and he surmised that my unusual quietness stemmed from worrying.

I had been worrying. I felt restless and impatient as I perceived our situation to be stalling out. One day in late July, the twins visited the zoo with their grandparents, and Rich was resting. At first I thought I would use the unexpected quiet time to unpack and organize the contents of the last few boxes, but a voice inside suggested that I reorganize my thinking instead. The worrying wasn't doing our situation any good, and it was a true indicator that I was trying to shoulder all of the problems.

As my thoughts continued along this path, I realized that, once again, I had succumbed to the faulty thinking that I had to do it all by myself. The worrying was a direct result of my fear of the unknown and of failure. Working from fear—a low-level, weakened state—was counter-productive. I had to work from strength. I always carried within me the ultimate source of strength and power to change my circumstances. When I allowed God's wisdom to source through me, everything connected to God's perfect energy. I had to get my incorrect thinking out of the way, focus on what I wanted to happen, and the how would be handled for me.

Why is this so hard? I silently yelled. For a moment, I admonished myself for allowing my thinking to get so far off track. I had already handed all of this over to God. Why couldn't I stay on target? Why was I trying to take it on again? But then, just as quickly, I realized that this self-recrimination was also faulty, useless thinking.

Okay, I told myself, *just let it go. Gratefully give it back to God and listen for the returned wisdom.* I immediately felt my spirits lift as I reconnected to God's energy. I thanked God for the present clarity of thought and also for sending the gift of wisdom, knowing it would be delivered at the perfect time and by the perfect means or messenger. I resolved to work harder to keep my thoughts more disciplined. When fear slipped back in, I would recognize its negative state and gently move my thoughts to the positive outcome I intended to create. *Today's a rehearsal for tomorrow,* I told myself, *and tomorrow I'll do a better job with the script.*

I slowly returned from my thoughts when I heard Todd and Ryan bustling in the door, already sharing tales from the zoo. I joined the twins and my parents in the kitchen, settling around the table for a snack as the stories unfolded. Rich wandered in a few minutes later and was soon caught up in the twins' noisy accounts of their animal sightings.

Later that evening, after observing many three-year-old renditions of lion roars and penguin walking, I finally tucked the twins into bed. Before heading to bed myself, I called my parents to thank them for the zoo outing with Todd and Ryan.

My dad answered the phone and said,

"Oh honey, I'm glad you called. In fact, I was just coming to the phone to call you. I've been looking through a stack of newspapers from Hutchinson that I hadn't found time to get to, and in the July 16th paper, there was an article about...," and he continued to share what he had just read. I was immediately enthusiastic, and Dad promised to explore the information further the next morning.

As promised, my dad made a phone call the next day and reported back to me. The article he had discovered was about a young man who had made an amazing recovery from MS. There was also a photo of him jumping beside the wheelchair he had formerly been confined to. Marvin had phoned the young man's stepfather, Bill Cole, someone Marvin had known when he lived in Hutchinson, Kansas. Bill was extremely helpful and encouraged us to get in touch with Vince, the young man from the article.

I barely contained my excitement as I relayed the information to Rich. He absorbed

Hutchinson News Wed., July 16, 1980

He gave up hope for faith

Hope is sometimes a thing that blinds, a mirage that appears on the horizon. And sometimes hope is just the thing to get you through the night.

But Vincent Stephens no longer has to hope. He believes.

He moves with a kind of halting jump in his step and to hold onto something he must clutch it tightly, but otherwise he's getting along just fine.

He's out of his wheelchair and he's back attempting to play his bass guitar. He's not looking forward to a gig with a rock band, but he is looking forward to getting married in September.

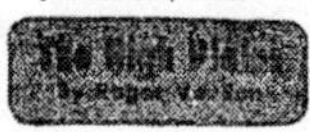

He's got multiple sclerosis but he's better than he was and he claims his diet made it so.

Eleven years ago he realized something was happening to his hands; he wasn't as agile as he once was. His guitar picking wasn't as quick or as exact. Something was wrong.

His condition was diagnosed as multiple sclerosis and he was given "ten minutes to two years to live."

By 1976 he was in a wheelchair, his speech impaired, his nerves unable to fully comprehend signals from the brain.

He visited doctors but there wasn't much they could do, he says. "The impression I got was 'enjoy yourself, it's down hill from now on.'"

Last week, for the first time in three years, he took a drink from a glass without the aid of a straw and without his arm jerking about uncontrollably.

His double-vision of three years has been cleared up for some time. Last January he got out of his wheelchair, went to a walker, and now gets around on his own steam — unaided.

He says doctors believe he is only enjoying a temporary remission. He doesn't care what they think.

He takes 32 pills twice a day.

The pills are vitamins and food supplements, including vitamins E, B-complex, C, calcium, alfalfa, lecithin, and others. He's also cut out his intake of white sugar, animal fat and gluten. He's cut his dosage from a daily intake of 128 pills a day to 64. "I'm into nutrition — very deeply," the 28-year-old says.

Although doctors have told him that his improvement is probably only a brief interlude before his full condition returns, Stephens says he's had brief remissions before: he's been able to control a fork for a week at a time.

His present "remission" has been ongoing and his condition has been improving since January 1979.

Mary Schnurr, an MS victim for the last 15 years, says Stephens "has improved a lot, he's surprising." She began taking a combination of vitamins and diet supplements herself last January and says she no longer feels tired or run-down and her balance is getting better.

"I think everybody that's got MS should try our little method," she says.

While Stephens is no medical expert, he knows what he knows. He knows how he can now walk, speak, and he can cook for himself and feed himself. The possibility that the medical experts are right still hovers over him. But his spirits are up and he believes he's found something worth sharing with others.

By getting others like himself involved in taking vitamins or diet supplements he could be doing himself a favor. He is a distributor for a firm which makes the pills he takes. He says he became a distributor so he could get his own supply cheaper ("I'm eating more profits than I'm making.") But he also says he doesn't care if people get the pills from him or from someone else.

He just wants to let people know he thinks he's come up with something — not a cure, by any means — but just something. If anybody wants to listen, fine. If the world turns a deaf ear to his door, that's fine too. Either way, his phone number is 669-1268.

Vincent Stephens has escaped the confines of his wheelchair. By Tom Bell the details with some reservation, not wanting to make too many assumptions from what little we knew. Rich agreed with me, though, that he should call Vince right away.

When Rich hung up the phone, I eagerly waited to hear his reactions. Rich appeared relieved and said, "Vince's coming. He's going to be in Colorado in a few weeks, and he said that he'd tell us the whole story then. He confirmed everything your dad told us. Sounds incredible!"

I arranged for the twins to play at my parents' house during the time of Vince's visit. Neither Rich nor I knew what to expect, yet neither of us were prepared for our first impression of Vince. When we answered the doorbell, a young man of medium height and build stood before us without any of the visible trappings of a man with MS.

Vince greeted us good-naturedly. I tried not to look too astonished as I directed everyone into the family room. Vince removed any awkwardness with his friendly smile and by addressing immediately what he saw in our faces. “It is amazing, isn’t it?” he began. “I couldn’t walk. I could barely talk. And now look at me!” he said as he opened his arms out to his side in an attitude of profound awe.

It was truly amazing! Rich and I couldn’t see any indication of the MS except for something slight in his speech and gait. How did he get from where he’d been to this? We hung on every word as Vince began to relate the details of his recovery.

Vince began his story at a seemingly hurried pace, as one remembering something painful and wishing to fast-forward beyond the hurting. He told us that his MS symptoms began when he was seventeen and a senior in high school. At first he noticed that he was unable to play the bass in the school orchestra and in his rock band with his normal level of precision. Next, he began to have tremors and numbness in his legs after athletic events. At this point, he became concerned enough to seek medical help. He discussed his symptoms with his family physician, and then he and his parents sought advice from a specialist in Wichita. After more than a week of intense testing, the specialist presented his diagnosis of an inoperable brain tumor and gave Vince two minutes to two years to live. A month later, Vince and his mom flew to the Mayo Clinic in Rochester, Minnesota, where the doctors negated the brain tumor diagnosis and delivered the MS diagnosis.

Continuing to talk rapidly, Vince recalled his immediate relief that the diagnosis hadn't been something as abruptly terminal as a brain tumor. He knew, though, that his diagnosis was bleak, so he had attempted to live as normal a life as possible for as long as possible. But it became progressively harder to do so. Over a six-year period, he transformed from a typically active, carefree teenage boy to someone who couldn't walk, couldn't feed himself, and could barely talk; he became an angry, depressed young man trapped in a wheelchair.

While Vince raced through these memories, he appeared to be staring at something beyond the window. I soon realized that his eyes were actually focused on mental pictures of his past. Then his eyes met mine, and I felt the lingering sadness from those images. He continued to share his story, but a little more slowly, as though losing energy from the pain of reopening his wound.

Vince remembered thinking, at the time, that his anger seemed justified considering his circumstances. But he directed his rage at the people who were trying to help. The more they tried to assist him, the more it fueled his self-pitying anger. Finally, though, Vince knew he had to make a decision. He could remain in this wallowing state, figure out an exit strategy from this life, or redirect the energy of his anger toward the disease and fight back.

Vince exhaled deeply and reconnected with the room. His whole demeanor began to shift as he repositioned his body. Where his shoulders had been tensed and his hands fisted, he now rested a more relaxed arm on his leg and released the tension from his fingers. A slight smile rose on his lips, and he held our gaze. He told us he had become frustrated and tired of blindly following the advice of the myriad doctors he had seen over the years. These doctors admittedly didn't know how to cure MS and had treated Vince with drugs that were supposed to either bring relief or reduce the severity of his symptoms. He intuitively suspected that even though the doctors were using all of their training and resources to try to help him, this course of treatment was actually doing more harm than good. He was ready for a new approach; the old one hadn't worked. And, as soon as he made this mental shift of attitude, his path to recovery began to reveal itself.

With the assistance of those who were caring for him, Vince looked for information related to successful treatments and recoveries from MS. The most encouraging articles were from England and Germany. Doctors and patients reported a high rate of recovery from MS when they altered their diets. They removed gluten, sugar, and animal fat. They also supplemented the diet with vitamins and minerals.

"And that's what I did," Vince said with an obvious air of determination. He then shared how he had replaced the gluten-filled breads and pastas—those made from wheat, barley, or rye—with products made from rice. He replaced sugar with honey and stopped consuming alcoholic beverages and sodas. He eliminated red meat and switched to chicken and fish. He started using low-fat milk, cut back on cheese, and sought organically grown fruits and vegetables.

Vince said none of this had been too difficult. He and his caretakers were still able to grocery shop at their local market, even though at first they had to carefully study labels to determine which brands of foods met the restricted requirements. Sugar and gluten turned up in the most unexpected places.

Once the appropriate brands were identified, though, the shopping routine resumed its normal time commitment.

The only problem with eliminating gluten, red meat, and most dairy products, he concluded, was that they contained essential nutrients. He then shared how his self-directed study produced a list of vitamins and minerals that were necessary for this altered diet. Next, he located a source of food supplements that would provide more vitamins and minerals to his diet and could be taken in large quantities without concerns of toxicity. "In fact," he shared with a grin, "at one point, I was taking almost 200 tablets a day!"

Rich and I listened intently as Vince continued. At first, he said, his improvement wasn't noticeable to others, but he could feel that he was better. Over a period of four years, though, he became strong enough to move from the wheelchair to a walker, from the walker to a cane, and finally to needing no assistance at all.

Rich and I looked at each other and then back to Vince. I spoke for both of us when I blurted, "That's it? You changed your diet and added the supplements. That's it? It sounds so simple!"

"Yes," Vince agreed, "that's it! But, it's also more than that. It's really more about attitude." He then continued to share the essence of his recovery. He said that when he finally decided to take charge of his own health, he had to retrain his thinking as well as the thinking of those around him. He realized that he was in charge of and responsible for his recovery, not the doctors or those who were caring for him.

"This idea of relegating our health care to someone else happens at a very young age," he said. "Think about how often someone handed you a pill or a spoonful of liquid every time you had something as slight as a cold. So as an adult, you automatically still followed the same pattern of expecting someone else to cure you. And when they didn't have a cure, you assumed there wasn't one. But it only meant *they* didn't know the cure; it didn't mean there wasn't one."

Vince said he thought he knew what had set him up as a target for MS. He believes he had significant but unknown food sensitivities for a long time. He probably always had some symptoms associated with the sensitivities, but he hadn't understood their connection. And by not understanding what these food sensitivities were, he'd been steadily abusing his body by eating and drinking the wrong things on a daily basis. Add this to his stressful lifestyle, and suddenly the door was open to disease. He didn't know why it was MS that had targeted him, but he thought that he probably had been a prime candidate for any number of equally devastating conditions.

Rich asked Vince, "Do you think you'll always need to stick closely to the diet changes and all the supplements?"

Vince cocked his head slightly to one side and replied, "I don't know. I can tell you at this point, though, that when I either purposely or accidentally eat or drink something I shouldn't, I have an adverse reaction that lets me know to get back on track. Maybe someday I won't have to be so strict about it, but I'm not even close to being there yet. It took me all those years of abusing my body by feeding it the wrong stuff to get into that wheelchair." He continued with a big grin, "It's taken me four years to get out of it, and I'll do whatever it takes to stay out of it! "

Then Vince looked seriously at Rich and said, "But don't do this because you think I'm telling you what to do. Do this only if you whole-heartedly want to do it for yourself. Figure out on your own what your body tolerates or doesn't. Try what I'm doing if you want, but also look at other possibilities. It's your choice. You're in charge!"

Vince continued to look directly at Rich and said, "You might also want to look at the other areas of your life that may have contributed to the decline of your health. Look especially at the stress makers and how you handled or didn't handle the stress. I was probably pushing too hard with my band gigs and car-racing hobby while my body was trying to deal with the effects of my wrong food choices. Think about what all you were pushing your body to do."

Rich and I exchanged a knowing look before returning our attention back to Vince.

Then Vince looked from Rich to me and voiced another suggestion. "Linda," he said, "consider how and when you offer support. It's important to help by putting together the healthy meals. It's also really necessary to let him know that you support his decision to get enough rest while he's recovering. He's probably going to need a nap each day in addition to a good night's sleep. Support his good decisions, but...don't baby him, and don't kill him with kindness. If he starts having his own pity party, get on him about it. Treat him as a normal person, and..." He paused for emphasis and then said, "Remember, it's his body. He's in charge."

Vince hesitated again and smiled, possibly considering whether to share scenarios of his support group, but then moved on and redirected his attention back to Rich. They continued to discuss more details of the supplements while Rich jotted some notes.

I took the opportunity to sit back in my chair, relaxing a little more into the cushions, and became the observer. Vince had mentioned his car-racing hobby, and this imagery played in my mind. I pictured these two young men as highly crafted race cars that required superior fuel for maximum performance. Give them less than premium grade and they knocked or shut down altogether.

Why, then, hadn't this fuel connection been considered before? Every human model usually filled up three times a day, and the correct fuel mixture was critical to engine performance. Why wasn't an analysis of fuel specifications part of our annual check-up procedures? Why was it casually assumed that every person's body could run efficiently on ordinary fuel? Wouldn't it make more sense to consider the needs of each one individually?

As Vince prepared to leave, my focus returned to the conversation. I could see obvious signs of hope shining in Rich's eyes, and I felt a tremendous sense of relief. Knowing Rich as well as I did, I was certain he would embrace this information and run with it. My spirits soared as I realized it was possible to take positive action against this dreadful disease. Vince was walking, talking proof that it was feasible. What a gift he was handing us; one that had been tried and successfully performed. Once again, I silently began to repeat *thank you.*

As we walked to Vince's car, Rich and I thanked him for delivering in person the miraculous story of his recovery. He told us that it gave him enormous pleasure to do so and said he'd check on us to hear our success story.

Later that day, Rich and I shared with my parents everything we learned from Vince. They were equally relieved to hear the details of Vince's recovery. Everyone encouraged Rich to immediately embark on the plan.

CHAPTER 5: MESSAGES

Fall 1980

LOCATING MY CAR KEYS, I called to Rich to let him know that I was ready to leave. I carefully eased my expanded silhouette behind the steering wheel, and Rich slid in beside me. As we headed to a previously scheduled appointment with an internist, my eyes traced the rugged profile of the Rocky Mountains and played connect-the-dots between freckles of fall's foliage. Dust played in the lower rays of sunlight. Grasshoppers snapped their leaving, and Canada geese honked their return.

Rich had seen the internist once before, shortly after our move. During his first visit, he and the doctor had quickly developed a trusting rapport. The doctor was fairly close to Rich's age and identified with the untimely end to Rich's dental career. He said there were some recently developed testing procedures for MS that looked promising, and he thought they would soon be available. The doctor reiterated, though, what others had said before. He said that even if they conclusively determined that it was MS, there wasn't anything he could do to help Rich other than to relieve any associated discomfort from the symptoms.

During this second visit, when Rich shared Vince's story and suggestions, the young doctor enthusiastically encouraged Rich to try it. "Go for it, Rich!" he said. "It definitely won't hurt you. Just be careful to select the correct type of supplements and increase them slowly in order to see how your body responds."

The doctor also added a personal endorsement for taking an active part in the healing process. "More people could improve their conditions if they would take it upon themselves to look for the reasons that their bodies are out of sync and then make the appropriate adjustments," he told us. "Especially if they make those changes right away. Too many times, people get discouraged if there isn't an instant get-well pill, and they adapt their lives to the disease rather than looking inside for a cause and cure." He continued, "Patients can increase their chances of success, even when there isn't a known treatment, if they work on improving their overall health."

Rich nodded thoughtfully and told the doctor, "I've just read a statistic in an article that indicates only fifteen percent of people are willing to make any significant changes to their lifestyle, even if they're told what to do to improve their health." The doctor agreed and encouraged Rich to be part of that fifteen percent. He also invited him to check in frequently to relay his progress.

After consulting with the internist, Rich and I discussed at length how to make the diet changes. We decided to eliminate the sugar, gluten, and fatty meat as Vince recommended. We also decided that Rich should cut back on all dairy products and eggs. In addition, we agreed that he should eliminate alcohol and caffeine.

We decided it would be easier if we were to change the way the whole family ate. Rich and I resolved to find appealing ways to serve fish and fowl at home, but to let the twins know that they were not restricted in any way when we took them out to eat. We knew that eliminating sugar from Rich's diet would not be all that difficult because, unlike me, he really did not have much of a sweet tooth. He generally ate desserts to be polite. And, because of Rich's fatigue and dizziness, he didn't seem to desire his usual evening cocktail very often. It was fairly easy to eliminate altogether.

Some items on the restricted list were more difficult to remove. Caffeine was one of them. Rich relished rich, strong coffee. We had read that it was best to eliminate caffeine gradually to prevent headaches from withdrawal.

We decided to slowly mix decaffeinated coffee with regular coffee until we could eliminate the caffeine altogether. Rich and I also struggled at first with how to restrict gluten for Rich, but we eventually decided it wasn't all that hard. We would use rice pastas for the whole family, but we would serve gluten-free, rice bread to Rich, while serving the rest of the family more readily available breads.

But then we reminded ourselves that this was not about being easy or difficult. This was about getting Rich's body back on track and giving it a fighting chance to overcome the disease. I recalled the support role Vince had encouraged me to assume. Given the level of lethargy that could settle in with the MS fatigue or to anyone suffering from the mental anxiety of disease, this role was critical to the success of the plan. We had always shared responsibility for all of our endeavors. We reasoned that we would find a balance of roles in this new arena as well.

The supplements were an extra challenge. Rich and I were so grateful to Vince for determining safe brands and dosage. The challenge, though, was the expense. Without a doubt, the supplements, when taken in the suggested quantities and frequency, would strain our already tight budget even more. But everything in life had a price, including good and poor health. And we were committed to following the plan exactly and determined to bring about the same successful return to good health.

Rich and I felt reenergized by focusing on success. We had seen Vince and his embodiment of that success. We could envision it once again for ourselves. There was just one area that still needed to be addressed. Vince had advised us to try to identify all of the factors that might have contributed to weakening Rich's immune system in addition to the probable food-sensitivity connection.

I thought there were multiple contributing factors to Rich's health decline. I recalled how

Rich had been taking antihistamines for the five years prior to the symptoms. His allergy symptoms had flared when we moved back to the Midwest. Rich had been controlling his symptoms with over-the-counter antihistamines. I thought that the dehydrating effect of the medications, along with the dehydration caused by all of Rich's caffeine consumption, might have made his body more susceptible to an illness. I knew he had not consumed enough water to counteract the dehydrating duo.

The other culprit, I thought, was stress. I wondered if each body had an unseen, fine-line indicator that registered safe and unsafe levels of stress for that particular body, like the tachometer of a car. Everyone's threshold for stress is different. I knew Rich was more of a risk taker than I. But I surmised that he had unknowingly ventured into his body's unsafe stress zone. He was trying to balance the time and energy he spent working to support his family with the amount of quality time he spent with us. Simultaneously, he was growing the patient base of his dental practice and supervising the construction of a new office building. As if that weren't enough stress, the nature of his business was inherently stressful. The majority of patients brought their own anxiety with them as they walked in the door of the dental office.

I guessed, understanding Rich as well as I did, that some of the patients' stress transferred to him because of his caring compassion for them. He also likely had conflicting feelings between his kind nature and the often unavoidable administering of pain associated with dental care. He wore rubber gloves and a surgical mask to protect himself from obvious communicable diseases, but he needed to protect himself as well from the not-so-obvious and stealthy side effects of transmitted stress. I felt that Rich's daily exposure to high levels of multifaceted stress definitely contributed to his health crash.

As I related my theories, Rich listened and added his own perspective and analysis. He agreed with me that his daily reliance on antihistamines and caffeine was possibly a factor to consider. Fortunately, with the change of climate from the move, some of the allergy symptoms had backed off and diminished the need for so many antihistamines. He also thought I accurately analyzed the contributors to his stress. However, both of my conclusions only related to what could be observed, and Rich realized that he needed to look deeper into his perceptions.

"It's all in the thinking," Rich said. "This is one of the most fundamental truths." He felt that this was the area that needed to be examined most closely for imbalance. If his thinking was not in tune with the reality he intended to create, then he had set himself up for failure. So, he needed to examine his core value messages, the ones that were placed there by his parents and their belief systems.

Rich shared with me that one of his messages said that if he worked hard enough, he could accomplish anything he wanted. He said, "Okay, that's true, but maybe working smarter is just as important, or maybe more important, than working harder." He said he would make a mental adjustment to that thought whenever he perceived it playing in his mind.

He told me that another of his core messages said that if he worked too hard, he probably would get sick. "Oh boy," Rich grimaced, "there's a message that needs adjusting." He said he would change the recording so that it told him to keep his work in balance by keeping joy in his work. Too much joyful work would not make a person ill. That thought led him to the perception that needed the most adjusting.

Rich recalled the message from his parents' belief statements about success. It had run so many times in his mind that he, before this moment, actually thought it was his own belief statement as well. The message equated ultimate success with working in the field of health care. He realized that his parents had revered their physicians and dentists, and they had placed this reverence for those career fields in Rich's value center. He realized then that all he had created was built on the shaky foundation of someone else's dream for him. He recognized that his career choice was determined by this mental message and was made from a sense of duty rather than joy. He said this core thought needed an absolute overhaul. First of all, it was too limiting to equate success with such a narrow spectrum of career choices. Rich realized that he valued the aspect of service to others rather than specific medical careers. Second, this message also needed to include the aspect of joy. A successful career choice was based on passionately providing service to others and feeling good about it.

Rich said he knew he needed to forgive himself for faulty past thinking and redirect his thoughts away from any useless self-reproach. Any judgments at this point were a complete waste of energy. His resilient message did not need any modification. It reminded him that it is okay to fall down, especially if one does a better job of walking or running after standing up again. It was up to him to reinvent himself with a revised belief system.

Once again Rich said to me, "It's all in the thinking." He told me his inner monologue would remain focused and full of gratitude for the information that God provided through Vince. By improving on the present, Rich felt certain he was already creating a better future. He would also stay mentally open to all possibilities. God provided the right people at the right time with the right information. Rich was determined to pay attention and listen for God's messages instead of dismissing them as random, coincidental thinking.

Both Rich and I viewed coincidental moments differently now than we had in the past. We formerly saw a coincidence as a random, yet usually fortuitous, event. Now, however, we viewed a coincidence as an opportune connecting point. This coinciding moment facilitated the perfectly timed, God-sourced conveyance of information from one person to another. When we actively watched for the coinciding events, we were more prepared to use the resulting messages as window-of-opportunity springboards.

Rich and I valued the opportunity to evaluate the past and learn from the experience. One major detour was enough. We knew that we should not dwell on the past events if we were going to move forward, however. Both of us realized the need to honor the past while, at the same time, detaching from it and the resulting illness. We knew we must focus entirely on the present challenges and opportunities.

We began our plan, as we did all of our adventures, by envisioning and discussing together what we intended to happen. We pictured Rich regaining his health, and we imagined him returning to a successful career. We did not know at that time whether the successful career would include dentistry. Sometimes, we concluded, ties to the past became weighted chains; we wanted to be open and unconditional. Together we poured our combined thoughts into creating a new dream.

Rich and I always tried to create big dreams. In fact, we believed if there was not a giggle factor in a dream, it wasn't big enough. A dream should be so enormous that it's almost laughable. Only a lack of imagination should limit the dream. The challenge was to recognize the link between dream and reality and watch for connecting opportunities. We imagined ourselves welcoming good health and unlimited abundance back into our lives, and we were both determined to bring this reality into fruition.

The changes were too subtle at first for those outside of the family to notice. But within two months, Rich and I knew we were on the right track, and the timing couldn't have been better. Halfway through November, I delivered a healthy baby boy. Rich felt well enough to be with me, as he had been for the delivery of the twins.

Todd and Ryan were delighted with their

baby brother. The twins, having recently turned four, naturally assumed the role of entertainers and protectors. I gratefully shifted my energy to caring for our newborn as the rest of the family prepared for the holidays. We had so much to be thankful for, and at the top of the list was our precious newborn, Jonathan, whose name means "gift of God."

CHAPTER 6: RESTORATION

Winter 1980-81

I ROCKED FROM ONE FOOT TO the other as I cradled Jonathan in my arms. Sunlight blanketed us in its warmth as it radiated through the window. I entertained him with an excited description of the mountainous winter splendor that lay beyond, and his intense stare appeared to take in every detail. Pointed mountain peaks and evergreens wore hooded cloaks of fresh snow. The high-altitude sun conjured icicles from tips of branches next to pinecone clusters. Redheaded finches sang carols of gratitude near our feeder. Stately, stepping deer paraded in reverent silence. Cars sporting ski-rack antlers carefully traversed the snowy streets.

Even with the arrival of our new baby and throughout the holiday season, Rich and I remained vigilant to our health-restoration campaign. By early January, we were certain that Rich's downhill slide was leveling off. No new symptoms had erupted, and those already present were beginning to subside.

By the end of January, shortly after his thirty-fourth birthday, I could tell Rich felt encouraged by a consistently stronger energy level. The heavy load of constant fatigue caused by the MS slowly released its grip. His fingers still felt numb, and there were still days he relied on the cane for support. But with each consecutive month, there was increased reason for celebration. Rich told me he felt certain his health was returning and it was time to begin the next steps toward a new dream. We both watched for connecting-point windows.

EPILOGUE

Spring 2004

A BIRD'S FLIGHT BRIEFLY interrupted the dancing stream of light pouring through the basement window. The slight movement was enough to return my attention to the task of sorting. I suddenly became aware of how long I'd allowed my thoughts to wander backwards. I shook my head slightly from side to side, laughed out loud, and redirected my thoughts to the object that had sent me on the mental wandering.

I distractedly found a safe place to rest my now-cold mug of tea and wrapped both hands around the wooden shaft of the cane. Dust diamonds sparkled in the window's brilliant light as I steadied the cane. Twenty-two years had passed since the cane had been needed. Rich had obtained a definitive diagnosis of MS in the spring of 1981. When he received the diagnosis, however, we were fairly certain that his recovery was already underway. By the spring of 1982, his health had completely returned, with the exception of partial loss of peripheral vision and numbness in the fingers of his left hand.

Rich followed Vince's plan exactly for three years, then he began to gradually reintroduce the foods that he had avoided during those three years. He successfully added some of the items on the restricted list, but he was never able to consistently consume sugar, most grains, dairy products, or eggs without adverse reactions. These specific food sensitivities had also been confirmed through more advanced medical testing. His continued good health and high energy levels were still closely tied to his efforts to honor his body's unique fueling requirements and maintain a better balance in his life.

Rich's revised core messages helped him discover an entirely new career in which he could still be of service to others, even with numb fingers. He retrained and created a successful career in real estate, followed by an even more successful career in mortgage banking. He found great joy in helping others realize their dreams while reaching his own. The possibility of making his dreams come true, including even those that made us giggle, always made life extremely interesting. He continued to enjoy a healthy, energetic, productive life.

I was able to stay at home with our boys until all three were in school. Then I returned to the classroom, earned my master's degree, and continued to teach until all three of our sons graduated from college.

Both Rich and I became better at understanding and interpreting our handling of the present and, in turn, how our present thoughts and actions affect our future. We improved at forecasting events and averting disaster by realigning our thinking or altering the belief messages beneath our thinking. Of course, there were still times we missed the significance of a connection or chose to ignore messages and windows. When misconnects occurred, we tried to remember to handle the challenge with a positive attitude, always looking for hidden gifts.

In one decisive movement, I dropped the cane on the pile destined for a charity organization. I hoped the next person who used it, like Rich, would need it for only a short while. I acknowledged, once again, the infinite gratitude I felt for the events and people who had come into our lives with the perfect timing to open the windows to our incredibly bright and abundant future. The blessings of knowledge and assistance continued to amaze and fill me with awe.

My thoughts then turned to the issues that had begun to tug at me: Why had we been given this gift of another chance to live life fully and abundantly? Was it merely because we had responded to the challenge, or were we supposed to allow the information to source through us to as many people as possible?

Of course, I reasoned, new diagnostic tools could now detect MS and other autoimmune diseases more quickly. And new drugs seemed to delay the disease's progression, and in some cases, even diminish the severity of its progression. But what about the people who aren't finding success with these drugs or are not satisfied with just delaying the devastation? What about those who would take the time to actively restore their health and abundance if they were just given the gift of a plan and the hopeful knowledge of its success?

At the first hint of a symptom, or the minute after a diagnosis of any autoimmune-related disease, people must to do everything within their power to support their immune systems. At the same time, they need to determine the reasons their bodies became susceptible to the disease and work to reduce and remedy the causes of inflammation in their bodies. They should immediately look into the possibility of altering and supplementing their diet. Finally, they should take the time to examine and amend, if necessary, their core value messages.

And what about their children, the genetically susceptible offspring? What about the "cluster" effect of autoimmune diseases within families whereby one person might have MS, another celiac disease, and another rheumatoid arthritis? The offspring may or may not be more at risk for an autoimmune disease, depending upon their own genetic make-up. However, because of the increased possibility, any allergy symptoms or signs of inflammation should be carefully evaluated rather than suppressed with medications. On an even more proactive level, diet modifications should be considered.

I also thought that there were people who, though generally in good health, experience allergy symptoms. They might attribute all their symptoms to airborne allergies, never suspecting that consumption of certain foods could be causing some of the inflammation and allergic reactions. There might be others who suffer from joint or digestive disorders and have not realized the connection between discomfort and food sensitivities. In all of these cases, already-stressed immune systems can be headed for a health crash if life's events serve up additional stress-filled challenges.

The intensity of my thoughts escalated as I recalled my role as supporter. I realized now with even greater clarity the importance of that role. Family and friends of someone newly diagnosed with an autoimmune disease need to realize that the person's possible denial and fatigue stand in direct opposition to intervention and recovery. Their supporting roles are critical to a successful plan.

I was certain that the tugging feeling I had been experiencing with increasing intensity was a message that it was time for us to share our information with more people. Over the years, Rich and I had told our story to people who were newly diagnosed with MS and to concerned relatives and friends. Now, I thought, it was time to deliver our gift of knowledge and hope to as many people as possible.

I wasn't sure how I would go about sharing the gift. I knew part of Rich's successful formula included his mental detachment from the disease, so I didn't want to involve him too much in the process. I paused for a moment longer then smiled to myself. I knew the answers would be given to me at the right time, and that the right people would come into my life to make it happen. I was certain of it now. I would be watching for the messages.

Q&A WITH LINDA AND RICH

Q *Why did you wait until now to write this book?*

A (Linda) It had everything to do with timing. A friend of many years contacted me with the news that one of her children was diagnosed with MS, and she asked if I would share with her what we had done to put my husband in remission. As I attempted to convey the information in an e-mail, I felt familiar feelings of inadequacy as I tried to condense the steps into a short message. The healing had taken place on so many levels, and it just didn't seem possible to explain it without acknowledging the importance of all those levels. At the same time, I heard that another longtime friend was failing from amyotrophic lateral sclerosis, a devastating neurodegenerative disease. I began to wonder if the steps we'd taken to curb the MS could have made a difference in this friend's struggle against ALS. When I voiced these concerns, messages arrived from several people suggesting I write our story. The other part of the timing had to do with hindsight. Advancements in research and recent test results finally connected most of the dots between what we had done in 1980 and our success. That hindsight understanding also allowed us to consider preventive steps for our children, who have increased genetic susceptibility to autoimmune-related disease. And, at this point, it became clear to me that our message needed to reach other families who have elevated risk for autoimmune disease. The time was right to help bridge the gap between nutritional research and the public. I was simply the messenger.

Q *With your hindsight knowledge, what steps would you suggest a recently diagnosed person take to stop the progression of MS?*

A (Linda and Rich) We would wage a counter-attack on a physical level to build the immune system and remove causes of inflammation in the body. First, we would look into the most current research on supplements that have been recognized for enhancing immunity, especially the research involving vitamin D. The Harvard School of Public Health Press Release (http://www.hsph.harvard.edu/press/releases/) titled "High Levels of Vitamin D In the Body May Decrease the Risk of Multiple Sclerosis" references a study that appeared in the December 20, 2006, issue of the *Journal of the American Medical Association.* According to the release, Alberto Ascherio, senior author of the study and associate professor of nutrition and epidemiology of HSPH, said, "The results of this study converge with a growing body of experimental evidence supporting the importance of vitamin D in regulating the immune system and suppressing autoimmune reactions, which are thought by most experts to play a key role in the development of MS."

Next, we would seek a supportive physician or nutritionist to assist in selecting the most beneficial supplements. Consider using intense nutritional supplementation through whole food supplements. We would also look online for Web sites that assist with this knowledge base. We highly recommend the informational Web site http://www.direct-ms.org/.

The DIRECT-MS Web site was "set up primarily to provide reliable, science-based information on the role that nutritional factors play in MS to allow those affected by MS to make an informed decision on whether or not to use nutritional strategies for managing the disease and preventing it from occurring in loved ones." Dr. Ashton Embry, a research scientist from Calgary, Canada, supplied the site with information he found when his son was diagnosed with MS in 1995. His son is now symptom-free.

On the DIRECT-MS Web site Dr. Embry and associates created, Dr. Embry wrote that he "discovered abundant scientific evidence that indicates that various nutritional factors potentially play major roles in the onset and progression of MS. Strangely, this information was not made available to persons with MS by doctors nor by established MS charities." We agree with Dr. Embry: a disconnect exists between current research-based knowledge relevant to nutrition and the general medical community. His Web site provides a wealth of information and links to research, testimonials, recommended nutritional strategies, lists of supplements, and MS-friendly recipes.

One incredibly important link on the DIRECT-MS Web site is to Dr. Loren Cordain's research. Dr. Cordain (http://www.thepaleodiet.com), who wrote the Foreword to this book and is a professor in the Department of Health and Exercise Science at Colorado State University, is author of numerous peer-reviewed scientific articles as well as *The Paleo Diet, The Paleo Diet for Athletes,* and *The Dietary Cure for Acne.* I (Linda) had the distinct privilege of meeting with Dr. Cordain to discuss his cutting-edge research as it relates to MS and other auto-immune diseases. Dr. Cordain and his associates published a scientific paper (see his Web site link to "Review article, Modulation of immune function by dietary lectins in rheumatoid arthritis") that outlines how diet may promote the development of rheumatoid arthritis, an autoimmune disease, in genetically susceptible individuals. Dr. Cordain believes a similar mechanism may also be involved in the pathogenesis of MS. Since publication of the paper on rheumatoid arthritis, Dr. Cordain and his associates have identified the specific hormonal gut receptor, the epidermal growth factor receptor (EGF-R), that allows transmission of gut antigens, proteins that set off the autoimmune response in the bloodstream. Dr. Cordain clarifies further by saying, "A number of common foods contain substances called lectins that can bind this receptor and thereby gain access into the bloodstream. Not only do the lectins bind the receptor, but they also bind various food and bacterial peptides, smaller parts of proteins found within the gut, and drag these chimeric particles into the circulation in a Trojan Horse-like manner. We believe that in genetically susceptible people, defined by their HLA haplotype, who may have been exposed to certain viruses in their childhood, this continual exposure to foreign antigens from the gut sets off the autoimmune response in which certain elements of the immune system, T-cells primarily, are no longer able to distinguish self from non-self and begin to destroy certain of the body's own tissues in a process known as molecular mimicry. Hence, the method to the madness of restricting certain foods is that these foods contain lectins that bind the EGF-R that allows foreign gut peptides access to the peripheral immune system."

Dr. Cordain suggests the following quoted food restrictions:

1) All wheat foods. Wheat contains the lectin wheat germ agglutinin (WGA) that potently binds the EGF-R and also binds virtually all bacterial cell wall proteins and a variety of dairy proteins. Other cereal grains, such as rye and barley, contain lectins that may also bind the EGF-R. Hence, restricting most cereal grains is recommended for recently diagnosed MS patients.

2) All beans, legumes, and lentils. Kidney beans, navy beans, black beans, and pinto beans contain a substance called phytohemagglutinin (PHA) that also potently binds the EGF-R and stimulates white blood cells, T-cells, and others to produce substances called integrins. The integrins allow white blood cells to leave the bloodstream and enter the specific tissue that is being destroyed by the autoimmune response. Soybeans and all soy products contain a lectin called soybean agglutinin (SBA) that also binds the EGF-R, as do virtually all other beans and legumes—hence the rationale for their exclusion. Peanuts, not a nut at all, are a legume and contain the lectin peanut agglutinin (PNA), which has been shown to rapidly cross the gut in humans, enter circulation, and promote an inflammatory response similar to other legumes.

3) Tomatoes. Tomatoes contain the lectin known as tomato lectin (TL), which also has been shown to rapidly enter circulation in humans. It seems not to produce an inflammatory response but rather an anti-inflammatory response. However, it is still capable of binding gut bacterial peptides and dragging them along with it into the bloodstream.

4) All dairy products. Milk is essentially the filtered blood of cows and, as such, contains most of the hormones found in the cow's bloodstream. Most of these hormones get destroyed by enzymes in the gut during digestion and therefore are not problematic. The exception is a hormone called betacellulin, which not only escapes the gut's proteolytic enzymes, but also binds avidly to the EGF-R. It is unclear if betacellulin provides access to the circulation for other milk proteins, as in the Trojan Horse mechanism. However, there is good evidence that WGA can bind milk proteins that maintain molecular mimicry with the myelin proteins in MS patients.

5) Egg whites. Egg-white protein is no simple protein, but rather a conglomeration of multiple proteins. Most problematic is the egg-white protein lysozyme. Lysozyme and the complexes it forms with other egg-white proteins can cross the gut barrier, since lysozyme contains a sugar that specifically binds EGF-R and allows these protein complexes to enter circulation. Because lysozyme can also bind gut bacterial cell walls, these peptides gain access to circulation via the Trojan Horse mechanism. Once the (lysozyme / egg-white protein / bacterial-cell-wall protein) complex gains access to circulation, it has the potential to activate the immune system in a process called three-way molecular mimicry. In genetically susceptible individuals, this process causes the immune system to lose the ability to recognize self proteins from foreign proteins in such a manner that the immune system ultimately destroys the body's own tissues.

Dr. Cordain recommends a diet of fresh fruit, vegetables, nuts, lean meats, fish, and fowl. In addition, he suggests restricting fiery spices and paying attention to research on vitamin D deficiency as it relates to MS. In one of his newsletters, Dr. Cordain discusses how excessive consumption of whole grain cereals impairs vitamin D metabolism (see newsletter link, May 15, 2006, Volume 2, Issue 1, at www.thepaleodiet.com). During the course of his research, Dr. Cordain also found evidence of the connection between stressful events and the onset of autoimmune disease.

We believe Dr. Cordain's findings provide insight into the reasons that the diet restrictions, supplement implementation, and stress management strategies we put in place all those years ago were an integral part of Rich's recovery. We gratefully applaud his tireless efforts and recommend following his diet for as long as necessary to reach and maintain a recovery mode.

Our suggestions, then, for halting the progression of MS mainly concern fine-tuning supplements and diet to fit the individual. The typical American diet doesn't work for everyone. Unknowingly, many of us have sabotaged our health by consuming foods or beverages that deplete, rather than enhance, energy and health. It takes some effort to rethink eating patterns and make the necessary changes, but it's well worth that effort. The other essential component to recovery and maintaining wellness is keeping the body hydrated. It seems like such an easy concept, but it's often one of the hardest things to do with consistency.

It's critical for someone who has been diagnosed with MS to support his or her immune system. More than likely, though, the diagnosed person won't have the energy or desire to follow through with all of this on his or her own. Hopefully that person will have a family member or friend who will jump in and assist with the information-gathering and initial changes.

Q *Would you suggest these same steps for halting and/or preventing the onset of other autoimmune-related diseases?*

A (Linda and Rich) According to the American Autoimmune Related Diseases Association (http://www.aarda.org/), there are more than 80-100 known autoimmune diseases and an additional 40 diseases that are suspected to be autoimmune-related. At this time, 50 million Americans suffer from autoimmune diseases, with rising prevalence, and women are more likely than men to be affected. Genetic susceptibility causes autoimmune disease to "cluster" in families—not as one particular disease, but as a general tendency to the autoimmune process and, consequently, different autoimmune diseases. For example, one family member may have autoimmune hepatitis; another, celiac disease; another, rheumatoid arthritis. Yet fewer than six percent of Americans surveyed in a recent AARDA/Roper poll could identify an autoimmune disease.

Given the scope of this health crisis, it's incredibly important to evaluate each family's medical history. If the family history includes autoimmune disease, then we would refer the family to The Best Bet Diet Group link at the Multiple Sclerosis Resource Centre Web site, http://www.msrc.co.uk, and the Best Bet Treatment link at the DIRECT-MS Web site. There you will discover informative discussions on the immune system as it relates to autoimmune disease, food sensitivity testing options, diet restrictions, and recommended supplements to enhance the immune system. We think anyone concerned with halting or preventing the onset of an autoimmune-related disease should consider following these suggestions along with investigating any other diet restrictions relevant to each specific disease. We have recommended The Best Bet Diet and supplements to our sons as a precautionary measure.

Q *What specific supplements and dosages were suggested for Rich?*

A (Linda and Rich) We selected the brand and followed the dosage routine Vince shared with us. The products were from Shaklee. We're not endorsing Shaklee over any other brand but, at the time, they were unique in their standards and qualities. Now there are many companies that create excellent supplements. As for dosage, it was suggested that Rich use the liquid form of Shaklee's multiple vitamin and mineral food supplement, called Vita-Lea, three times a day with meals. It was also felt, at the time, that the liquid form would allow for better absorption. It's important to note that this was a whole-food supplement instead of a synthetic supplement. Because it was a whole-food supplement, Rich and Vince were able to take it several times a day without reaching toxic levels of certain vitamins, as might have been the case with a synthetic supplement. Additionally, Rich took a 500 mg vitamin C supplement with each meal and a vitamin B complex. At that time, vitamin C was beginning to be acknowledged for its antioxidant properties, and the vitamin B complex was recognized as support for the nervous system. We were very fortunate to have even the limited resources that were available to us in 1980. The advancements in the knowledge base and in the supplement industry have been incredible, making it a lot easier now for a newly diagnosed person to obtain high-quality supplements specifically designed to meet his or her needs.

We now know the supplements actually worked in tandem with the removal of the food and beverage items that were causing the problems. We removed sugar, most grains, fatty meat, caffeine, and alcohol from Rich's diet. We also restricted dairy products and eggs. Fortunately, legumes were rarely part of our meals at that time. By removing most of the troublesome components from his diet, we created a better environment for the absorption of the supplements and other food nutrients. This tandem effort, in turn, enhanced his immune system.

Q *Do you think everyone diagnosed with MS can benefit from the steps you've suggested?*

A (Linda and Rich) Just as we think each person has a fine-line indicator that determines acceptable and unacceptable levels of stress and inflammation, we also think each person has a unique timeline that gauges ability to recover from illness. Vince and Rich were both experiencing devastating symptoms, but both almost fully recovered from those symptoms. They obviously were given the information at the right moment and wholeheartedly embraced the steps to recovery. We don't know at what point either of them might not have been able to recover. We're not medically trained in this area, and our suggestions are not intended to replace a professional's advice and/or treatment. Our intention and hope is to relay this gift of information to those who will seize the opportunity to participate actively in restoring their health. Certainly, the sooner a person begins the process, the better the odds for full recovery.

Q *Why do you think these steps could help people recover from other illnesses or avoid illness all together?*

A (Linda) I realized the common link of inflammation to disease when I read *The Perricone Prescription* by Dr. Nicholas Perricone, M.D., 2002, Harper Collins, New York, NY. Dr. Perricone says, "I knew what I saw and never let it go. I continued to believe that inflammation was at the root of cancer and other acute and chronic diseases. Whenever I looked at a disease under a microscope—everything from arthritis to heart disease—inflammation was always a component. Every disease I studied had a common theme, whether it was cancer or aging: inflammation was present. I was convinced that inflammation was not simply a secondary response. I believed inflammation to be the key to the whole process of disease of every type."

This information helped us locate the last few pieces of the puzzle to understand the links between what we had done and Rich's recovery. It also helped connect the dots relating to my own stage-three melanoma cancer diagnosis in 1995. Until recently, I couldn't see the similarities. Now, with hindsight understanding, I see clearly the same progression of mistakes. I took over-the-counter or prescribed decongestant/antihistamines for sinus congestion and headaches, which contributed to dehydration. Early testing linked the allergies slightly to airborne sources, but at the time, food sensitivity testing was admittedly poor. My recent testing, however, has shown I have high sensitivity to dairy, eggs, and gluten. So, at the time of the illness, my immune system was struggling to deal with years of allergic reaction inflammation and poor digestion caused by consuming large amounts of dairy, eggs, and gluten. Then I unknowingly added unacceptable levels of stress to my body. I had set myself up for an illness by unwittingly causing diet-related inflammation and lack of nutrient absorption and then topped it all off with a large helping of too much stress; the same sequence of mistakes created, once again, the perfect environment for an illness. I think large numbers of illnesses probably follow a similar progression. Many people have already set themselves up for disease, and many people have unknowingly begun the process. I hope they'll hear about this recipe for disease and stop the progression of events before the onset of a devastating illness.

Q *Isn't it difficult to maintain such a restrictive diet?*

A (Linda and Rich) Yes and no... We would love to be able to eat everything we want *and* in any quantity! Who wouldn't? But we make the choice to feel well and live full, healthy, productive lives. Of course, it took time and self-dicipline to get beyond the craving stage for certain foods, or in Linda's case, for sugar! But, once we adjusted our diet to include only items that enhance our health and energy, we could tell very quickly when we'd eaten something we shouldn't have. Either the allergy symptoms turned on again, or we became sluggish, often with an upset stomach or headache. Now that we've become accustomed to feeling great all the time, it makes it a lot easier to avoid the food items that we've learned to associate with feelings of discomfort.

Q *You've talked about the physical level of steps you would suggest. Are there other levels?*

A (Linda and Rich) We talked about the physical level first because it's the most important to stopping the progression of the disease by waging an all-out counterattack. The other levels—the emotional and intellectual levels—must be addressed as well, but they're more about learning to control stress in order to remain healthy. We suspect most of our bodies are strong enough to take the abuse of inadequate diets and too much inflammation until stress-overload enters the picture. It becomes the "last straw." Our bodies are designed to recognize and ward off all sorts of diseases. But, when stress comes along, the troops patrolling the borders of the body are too few. Not only are our bodies dealing with inadequate nutrition and/or inflammation, but they're also trying to support organs under duress from stress. Suddenly, a virus encountered somewhere along the way has an unguarded entrance to an overly-taxed, malfunctioning immune system. Learning to recognize our individual limits of stress is critical to remaining healthy. We spent a lot of time reading other's comments on the subject while we reframed and reprogrammed our mental messages. And, it's definitely an ongoing process. The other level of understanding is to recognize the greatest source of wisdom through our spiritual connection with a God of our own understanding. This higher power's inspiration and creativity links us perfectly with whatever we need. It's up to us to be aware of those links and to watch for them.

Q *What would you say to diagnosed people who feel medications are working for them and don't want to make lifestyle changes?*

A (Linda and Rich) We would say we're really happy medications are working and have diminished their symptoms. We think that's wonderful. But, they may be lulled into a false sense of wellness. The medications are only buying them some time, because they're not really contributing to restoring health or dealing with the root causes of the disease. The medications are merely working to reduce and/or slow the progression of the symptoms. We think it's shortsighted not to feel that lifestyle changes need to be made. We think diagnosed people should feel, instead, a sense of urgency to gather as much information as possible about how to support their immune systems, remove the dietary and other causes of their inflammation, and reduce stress. It takes time and effort to make the changes, and some of those changes might be as hard as some of ours were to make. But, if those changes restore health and the ability to live life fully, it'll be well worth every bit of that time and effort.

Q *Rich, how are you doing now?*

A I'm fantastic! I've tried several times throughout the years to reintroduce the foods from the "avoid" list, and each time it resulted in a weakened immune system. Finally, I just gave up on trying to re-incorporate those food items. I still honor the diet restrictions on a fairly strict basis and find it a small price to pay for such an incredibly healthy and productive life!

Q *Have you spoken recently with Vince?*

A (Linda) I called Vince to see how he was doing and to see if he had time to review this writing project for me. When I asked how he was, I loved hearing his answer of, "Better than ever!" He isn't involved with racing cars any more, but he has a very active career and lifestyle. He still honors his unique dietary restrictions, although not as strictly as he did while he was recovering. We will be forever grateful to him for sharing his gift of information with us.

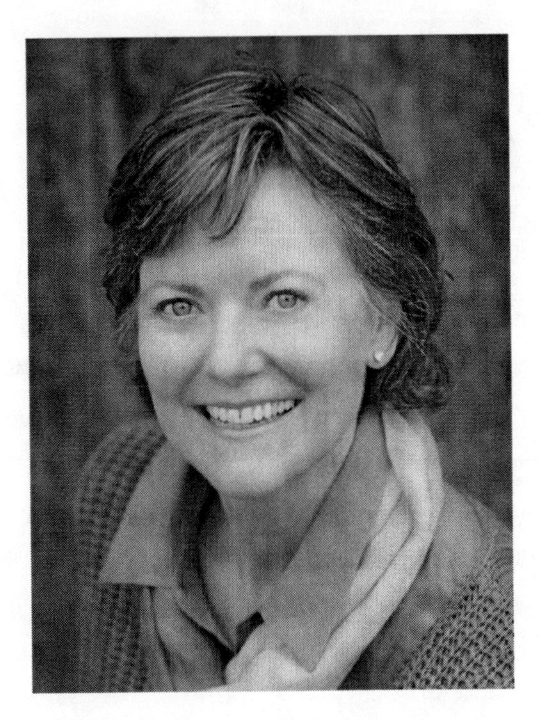

ABOUT THE AUTHOR

Linda Sollenberger Land earned a B.S. in Education from the University of Kansas and a Masters of Education from Lesley College. She is now retired from a teaching career that spanned 30 years. Linda enjoys traveling, hiking, and reading.